YC

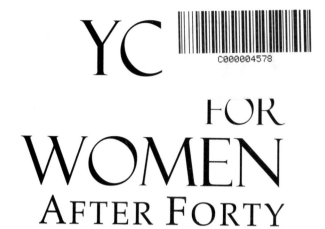

FOR WOMEN
AFTER FORTY

SEEMA SONDHI

wisdom
tree

To my mother who guided me lovingly

Cover model: Sharon Lowen
Photographs: Hemant Chawla

ISBN 978-81-8328-001-3

Published by
Wisdom Tree
4779/23, Ansari Road
Darya Ganj, Delhi-110002
Ph. 011-23247966/67/68
wisdomtreebooks@gmail.com

Printed in India

Preface

The middle age is a critical and an important stage in a woman's life, which is full of tremendous changes and if you are heading towards it you will feel that you just don't know yourself anymore. You are not the same active, confident office manager or the home manager you used to be; you find yourself thinking, talking and behaving in a totally different way. When you are in such a fragile and sensitive condition, yoga comes to the rescue and helps find the REAL YOU, which is hidden behind a veil of problems.

Regular practice of yoga *asana* with patience and dedication will transform you into a supple and flexible person, which means that in due course of time you can forget about the backaches, stiffness and the depression, increase your self-confidence and have a perfect body which you always desired.

Pranayama and meditation are closely linked. These methods strengthen the bond between your sub-conscious and the conscious mind and aid in healing the body, the mind and the spirit. They will instill a deeper sense of happiness, contentment and love for you.

Learn to accept the fact that you've done your bit as a daughter, friend, wife and mother. That though your body is slowing down, you as a woman have become wiser and stronger. Let yoga help you in this turbulent stage and take you closer to spirituality, towards the Divine who resides in your heart and in your body, in the scared shrine within you.

Contents

1

Yoga for Total Health

Yoga is a powerful tool and benefits women at all stages of life; it eases the pain of pre-menstrual syndrome as well as helps ease discomforts of pregnancy, childbirth and certain changes associated with menopause; it lowers risks of heart disease, high blood pressure and strokes; it benefits the body and mind by bringing in energy and balance in the body. The techniques of *asanas*, *pranayama*, relaxation and meditation help in creating strength in the internal body like the nerves, heart and adrenals glands and at the same time release all the negative emotions from the mind. The physical, spiritual and psychological aspects of yoga make it a useful therapy for all the ailments that women suffer at this stage of life. Yoga builds strength and improves flexibility in the muscles; it is good for the spine and releases all toxins from the spine and makes it supple. Through regular yoga practice, women can alleviate all the menopausal symptoms. Yoga helps to regulate and balance the metabolism and lets your body's natural wisdom determine your appropriate weight. *Pranayama* helps in the control of the breath and calming the mind. Through meditation we experience the inner stillness and peace;

above all, it helps us to connect spiritually as this is the deeper value and aim of all yoga practice.

The benefits of yoga are so profound that soon after the first session you will feel more relaxed, the overall muscles tone will improve, the spine will become strong and flexible improving all the systems of the body, like digestion, skin texture, intake of oxygen in the lungs, and providing better sleep. The immune system will strengthen and you will experience a sense of confidence in yourself, preparing you to face the challenges of the new life with love, respect and trust in yourself.

2

Yoga—Spiritual Practice

Yoga is the mind and body work-out which originated in India many centuries ago. Since then many have and are still enjoying the profound benefits of yoga. It connects the breath to the body and the mind to the muscles; it is more than just a physical experience; it works on the subtle parts of the body and mind resulting in quieting the distractions of the mind and building a healthy body.

In India the sage Pantanjali compiled the yoga *sutras*, or the eight steps to spiritual enlightenment.

Yama is the ethical conduct involving non-violence, truth, honesty, moderation and non-covetousness. *Niyama* is the moral conduct, positive self-action, purity, contentment, discipline, self-study, and self-surrender. *Asana* (yogic exercises) means finding a comfortable and a stable position. *Pranayama*, the art of *yogic* breathing by observing the breath and slowing down the breathing process, helps to master the body and still the mind. *Pratyahara* is the drawing of the mind's focus away from the external senses to the inner sensations of the body. When the mind is drawn inwards, then comes *dharana*, which helps to fix the mind on a single object, the breath or a *mantra*.

This is where *dharana* practice becomes very challenging as it is very difficult to focus or concentrate on a single object to the point of being completely absorbed in it. Then follows the next step—*dhyan* or meditation. When the mind is absorbed in meditation, all thoughts disappear and the mind stills leading to the final step—the *samadhi* (bliss and enlightenment) where everything melts into a feeling of oneness.

Let us take you on this *yogic* journey to discover the perfect harmony in your body and mind. Remember that it is through the eight limbs that you cultivate a steady mind and body to reach your goal.

3

Paths of Yoga

Yoga is an ancient science with a clear understanding of health and it honours all aspects of our inner being. It is a practice that encourages us to go within so as to connect you to your inner wisdom, your inner self. In yoga philosophy, there are four paths to attain this knowledge.

Karma yoga is a path of selflessness by serving and working without desiring an end reward. This is done without the desire of any personal gain and through the path of dedication, as by renouncing the fruits of one's actions. The action thus becomes unselfish. *Bhakti* yoga is worship of the Divine spirit, and is the path of devotion and love; chanting prayers and *mantras* is part of this path. This path is the easiest form of yoga to practice because we all possess the capability to love. With regular practice of *bhakti* yoga we can get rid of all our emotions and develop the highest virtue of love, evoking it from the depth of our inner self. *Jnana* yoga is the study of the self through spiritual scriptures; it is the intellectual approach to spiritual evolution. We learn to discriminate between the real and the unreal through the right inquiry and constant self-analysis. The mind is used to examine its own nature.

Raja yoga is a scientific and a systematic path of analysis, through meditation, and special techniques are used to understand the mind and ways to control it. It systematically erases ego, with the thinking mind and ego dissolving into oneness. *Raja* yoga is called the 'royal path' to attain the state of unity with mind, body and soul.

All these paths can be combined in *hatha* yoga to deepen the practice and spiritual connection. Practise *raja* yoga by drawing the awareness inward, focusing the mind on the breath and becoming still and meditative in the posture, then applying *karma* yoga by letting go of the need to reach anywhere. Simply do the posture without expecting any rewards from your practice. Make each posture a prayer, celebration of life, and invoke the power of *bhakti* to bring the energy of the Divine within you. Explore and become aware of the body and breath, using *jnana* yoga to study your body and the mind in posture. Practising yoga with full awareness will connect you spiritually and the results will be very enriching.

Understanding Menopause

Menopause like puberty is a critical and important stage in a woman's life. The term is self-explanatory as it literally means the 'pause' in a woman's menstrual cycle. It is a natural aspect of ageing and occurs in all women between the ages of 40 to 60 years. It occurs when the ovaries stop producing hormones called 'oestrogens'. This causes the oestrogen levels to drop, leading to the end of the monthly cycle. We must remember that menopause can occur earlier too if a woman's ovaries have been removed surgically for any reason.

Oestrogen is commonly known as the female hormone because it plays a key role in shaping the female body and preparing it for female functions, such as pregnancy, development of breasts for feeding infants. Above all, the uterus, the vagina and other female organs depend on the presence of oestrogen in the female body aiding in its development.

Progesterone is the second most important female hormone produced by the ovaries. This hormone helps in stimulating the growth of the cushiony lining the uterus where the fertilised egg grows and develops into a baby. It also helps the breasts to produce milk and generally sustains a pregnancy.

Together with progesterone, oestrogen regulates the changes that occur with each monthly period and prepares the uterus for pregnancy. Prior to menopause, the ovaries produce 90 per cent of oestrogen, while the other organs like the adrenal glands, liver, and kidneys also manufacture small amounts of this hormone. Due to the effect of low oestrogen level, a woman's skeletal system and the heart get affected besides leading to breast cancer and rendering the body weak generally.

All women suffer from troublesome symptoms during menopause, but the severity and frequency of these symptoms varies from woman to woman. The most common symptoms are:

Irregular bleeding: Changes such as a shorter or longer duration of period, heavier or light menstrual bleeding, and varying of time between periods may be the early signs of the onset of menopause.

Hot flashes: This is the most common symptom in menopause. A hot flash produces a sudden sensation of warmth or even intense heat in various parts of the body, especially the chest, face, and the head. Some women feel an increase in heart beats. The hot flashes may last for a few seconds or for several minutes.

Vaginal thinning: Oestrogen plays a key role in maintaining the functions of a woman's vagina and the surrounding tissues, the uterus, the urinary bladder, and the urethra. Since these organs may weaken or shrink, involuntary leakage of urine, infection, or painful urination are very common symptoms. Vaginal dryness and thinning occurs over a passage of time. Many women suffer from urinary incontinence and this invariably goes undiagnosed, as the women who suffer from it are too embarrassed to talk about it. But with regular practice of yoga techniques, like *mulabandha*, women can be helped considerably.

Osteoporosis occurs when the bones begin to lose their strength and density because of calcium loss. The bones become fragile and tend to fracture very easily. The word 'osteoporosis' literally means 'brittle bones'. It is often taken to be an old person's condition, but the truth is that more than one in every two women develops osteoporosis during middle age, especially after menopause when the hormone important to bone health is not produced by the body. We do not have control over some of the risk factors for osteoporosis, but we can create a lifestyle that prevents damage to the bones and maintains their condition. *Yogic* techniques such as *asanas*, breathing and mediation provide the best hope for minimising the effects of this disease or even preventing it altogether. *Yogic asanas* improve muscle strength, build bone density and improve glandular function. Yoga creates a balance between the ovaries, adrenals, parathyroid, pituitary and pineal glands and ensures that the body receives a steady supply of the right hormones for maintaining the bone strength and health of the entire skeletal system. Yoga improves the body posture and coordination, strengthens the muscles, increases flexibility and maintains balance.

Modern science has developed a cure for osteoporosis and that is the Hormone Replacement Therapy (HRT) which is based on the scientific knowledge that during menopause, a women's ovaries stop making the female hormone called oestrogen, thus causing unpleasant symptoms in the body. By prescribing oestrogen tablets to women, some of the symptoms could simply vanish. But, in reality, HRT does not cure the body of all the systems except for providing temporary relief. The symptoms return once the treatment is stopped. Further, HRT therapy is believed to cause side effects like cancer of the breast, uterus or the ovaries, and heart disease. But if women practise yoga regularly, all the symptoms stated above will vanish.

Heart disease: The incidence of heart disease rises considerably in women after menopause. Oestrogen can lower the high levels of bad cholesterol and help maintain healthy veins; it also lowers the blood pressure and maintains the blood sugar in the body.

Mood swings: The brain also responds well to oestrogen as it affects women's memory besides helping in healthy functioning of the nerves cells. Depression may set in during this phase of life.

Palpitations: This is another problem of the nervous system that women experience—it is as if the heart begins to beat like a thunder and this is due to a nervous reaction of fright and nothing else.

For most women, the symptoms of menopause last for a relatively short time. But the levels of oestrogen naturally remain low after menopause, affecting the body. Eating right and regular practice of yoga can help the woman to bring positive changes in her life.

5

Yoga, the Natural Healer

It is believed that every human being reflects his or her own energy field, a definite 'aura' around him or her, carrying with it an emotional energy created by his or her own internal and external experiences, which could be positive or negative. Every thought that you get in your mind creates energy and converts into matter. Remember that you are what you think you are, and so it becomes very important to understand to harbour thoughts which will nurture the body and the mind, as these two are interconnected. The mind and body cannot be separated from each other but it is necessary to unite them through daily practice of yoga.

A woman's body undergoes a series of physical and mental changes at puberty, pre- and post-pregnancy to menopause. Hence, it becomes very important for a woman to take to yoga—a 'natural system of exercise that will aid in healing the body faster during all phases of life. Started as a spiritual discipline, the practice of yoga has become a powerful remedy for all the ailments, ranging from menstrual cramps to rashes, from mood swings to varicose veins, making yoga a powerful healing tool for women. Healing in yoga is induced with direct participation by you where you are required to heal the mind and body consciously. Healing occurs in course of time according to each individual's practice or *sadhana*. Unlike the typical exercises that are available to women in the gymnasium which make the external muscles tight, yoga gives importance to the internal organs such as heart, lungs and the mind, creating a sense of well-being and at the same time giving you a healthy body.

The physical, spiritual and psychological aspects of yoga make it a useful therapy for all health ailments. It builds one's strength and improves flexibility by stretching the muscles. It is an excellent tonic for the spine as it loosens the spine and tones the entire nervous system. Regular practice of yoga *asanas* and *pranayama* strengthens the body and regulates the energy in the seven vital energy points or *chakras* by activating these energy points and freeing the body of all physical and psychological ailments. Yoga also counteracts negative emotions, such as anger, anxiety and depression provided you observe strict discipline and participate actively and positively to create a balance in the body, mind and spirit.

6

Asanas

Yoga exercises are called yoga *asanas* or postures and it is a well-known fact that with the regular practice of yoga *asanas*, the entire body is benefited while various menopausal symptoms are alleviated. Yoga postures are gentle and every woman can practise them, irrespective of the fact that they may have never done yoga before. *Asanas* are postures to be held, rather than exercises, and are performed slowly and meditatively, combined with deep abdominal breathing. These gentle movements not only reawaken your awareness and control of your body but also have a profound effect spiritually. At the end of each session you will feel relaxed and full of energy. Women who suffer from chronic back pain, insomnia, stiffness and depression benefit tremendously from the practice of yoga.

Those of you who have never practised yoga *asanas* before or are convinced that yoga is not for you, then keep a moment aside to ponder over its importance. It is the oldest spiritual art form and people from all walks of life practise yoga. A regular practice of yoga postures is very important for woman at this period of time, as it will induce relaxation, lower stress and relieve tension. The yoga postures have a profound effect on the physical and internal body besides

13

having an immeasurable effect on the entire endocrine system, including the pineal, pituitary, thyroid, parathyroid, and adrenal glands. Let it be noted that it is the endocrine glands that control the changes in hormonal levels during menopause. *Asanas* balance the endocrine system and raise the levels of endorphins that are involved in the body's positive responses to stress. The weight-bearing postures make the bones strong and improve the efficiency of the heart, making the heart strong.

Pranayama helps in the control of breath and in calming the mind. Through meditation we experience inner stillness and peace. Above all, it helps us to connect spiritually with the Divine as this is the deeper value and aim of all yoga practice.

Yoga Sutra defines *asana* as that posture which is comfortable and easy, as well as firm. It is a dynamic position, in which the practitioner is perfectly poised between activity and non-activity. A corresponding mental balance exists between movement and stillness with each posture reflecting a mental attitude. The forward bends make one strong and help in accepting the changes occurring in the body through an attitude of self-surrender. Backward bending postures assist in removal of fear, helping you move ahead in life with grace and dignity. Inverted postures relax and calm the body and help the body counter the hot flashes as they have a dramatic effect on the flow of blood to every organ of the body. They affect the endocrine system, pineal, thyroid, parathyroid and adrenal thus creating a balance in the body by regulating the flow of the hormonal changes. Standing postures help you to become emotionally strong and help you focus on your goal of loving and caring for yourself.

7

Let's Get Started

Remember, whatever your size or shape, you can enjoy these relaxing and invigorating yoga *asanas* that benefit the heart and bones, regulate your weight, sculpt your body, improve your concentration, boost your immune system and enhance your memory. Anybody can practice yoga; you do not need any special equipment or clothes—just a small, quiet space and a yearning for a healthier, quieter life. Regular practice of yoga renders your body fit and beautiful, increases your energy and vitality, reduces stress and increases your powers of concentration and discipline.

If you have never practised yoga before, you will need to follow some simple but important guidelines to get the most of benefits out of your yoga sessions.

Find a suitable, well-ventilated room. Try to set aside a specific time each day for your yoga session.

A sticky mat is the perfect surface for yoga postures because it keeps your feet, hands and elbows from slipping, allowing you to stretch to your full potential. Yoga mats also provide a small amount of padding, just enough to keep knees and elbows from bruising.

- Do not eat anything for two hours before the yoga session.
- Dress in loose, comfortable clothes, preferably cotton, as your body needs to breathe during your sessions. Leave your feet bare and remove your watch or any jewellery that you may be wearing.
- Put on some light music, as it will be soothing and help you to take your mind off the discomfort you may experience during stretching.
- Remember you don't have to be thin, trim and lean to practise yoga. Change the yoga postures to suit your figure condition and weight.
- Start with a few minutes of gentle movements and then deepen your practice. Never ever force the body to do postures it finds difficult to adopt. Use support, such as cushions, blankets, bolsters and straps to support your body during your yoga practice.
- Become aware of past injuries or arthritic condition and move into posture very gently. Work on maintaining the body; flexibility will be the side effect if your regularly practise.
- If you run short of breath or when the body fights to breathe, it is a sign that you are going past your body's capacity.
- Maintain a healthy attitude and not that of competition; do not give importance to the results. Try and hold the posture for as

long as the body feels comfortable, and practise on your own pace. Never jerk or strain your body while doing the *asanas*.

- Try to rope in friends so that you have company and get motivated to continue your practice.
- If you are not confident to start the practice on your own, join a yoga centre and later continue to practise on your own.

Surya Namaskar (Sun Salutation)

Surya namaskar is an important part of yoga practice. It is a series of 12 continuous postures that are practised in a flowing series. It is always good to begin the yoga session with a few rounds of *surya namaskar* as it stretches all parts of the body muscles; it generates heat, warms the muscle tissues and helps the body to become flexible while protecting the body from any injury. It is also a very good cardiovascular exercise and improves the circulation of blood throughout the body.

Surya namaskar improves the overall body strength and builds a person's stamina.

As a few of you would have never done yoga before. You may find the sun salutation a little demanding on the body, so we suggest a kneeling down *surya namaskar* which can be easily adapted by everybody.

Let's start:
Begin by kneeling down on the floor and placing the hips on the separate heels. Keep the arms on the thighs with palms facing the thighs, maintaining the spine and neck straight. Close your eyes and become aware of your whole body. Begin to relax your body mentally.

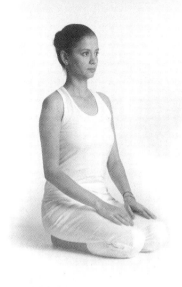
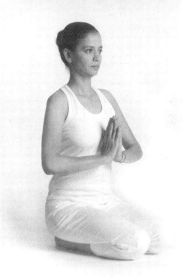
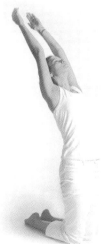
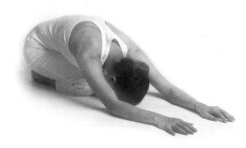

19

- Exhale. Join your palms together in a *namaskar* position in front of your chest and mentally pay your respects to the sun-god by saying mentally, *Om surya namah*.

- Inhale. Stand on the knees, stretch your arms straight up over your head or place the palms behind the back for support, arching your body backwards.

- Exhale. Slowly bend forward, bringing your palms to the floor and touch your forehead to the floor.

- Inhale. Without moving your hands, lift the head and hips while arching the spine down.

- Exhale. Tuck the toes in and without moving the hands and the feet, lift the hips and lower the head between the arms so that the body forms a triangle.

- Retain your breath. Dip your knees, chest and forehead to the floor; if this is difficult initially, then lower your knees first, then your chest and finally your chin. Then move your hips up.

- Inhale. Slide your body forward till your hips are on the floor. Arch your back and chest upward and drop your head back. Your legs, hips and hands remain on the floor.

- Exhale. Tuck your toes in and without moving your hands and feet, lift your hips as high up as possible. Lower your head between your arms so that your body forms a triangle.

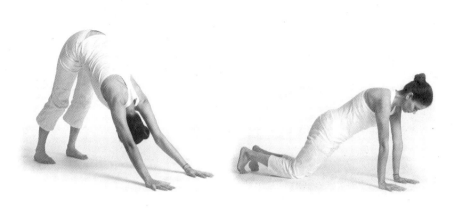

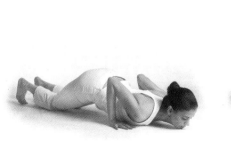

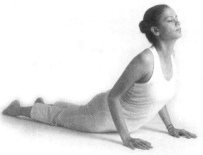

21

- Inhale. Drop the knees down and without moving the hands, lift the head and hips and arch the spine down.
- Exhale. Without moving your hands, slowly place the hips on the ankles and touch the forehead on the floor.
- Inhale. Raise the body up and stand on the knees. Stretch your body up and arch backwards.
- Exhale. Bring both the palms together in a *namaskar* at chest level.
- Relax.
- These 12 positions are practiced once to complete one round of *surya namaskar*.

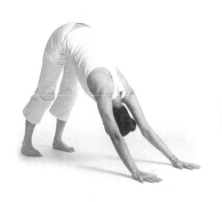

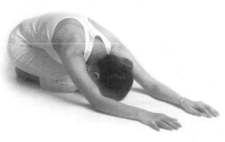

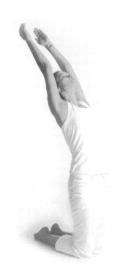

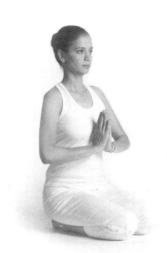

Tadasana (Standing Pose)

The entire spine is stretched in this pose, toning the spinal nerves; it stretches the abdominal muscles and releases all the stiffness on the shoulders. This *asana* also develops mental balance.

- Stand with feet together, toes, ankles and arms by the side. Distribute the weight of the body equally on both the feet, tighten the knees, and gently contract the hip and abdominal muscles, pulling the chest out and with neck held straight.

- Inhale. Raise both the arms up and stretch the entire body. Hold the posture for a few seconds.

- Exhale. Release the posture by bringing the arms down.

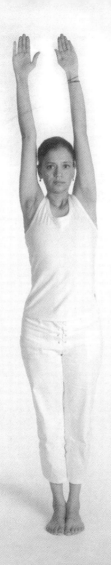

Tiryaka Tadasana (Standing Side Stretch)

This posture benefits the waist, arms, and fingers and releases all the stiffness in the back and the postural muscles.

- Stand with feet together or 10 cms apart, arms by the side and head straight. Close the eyes and steady the body.
- Inhale, raise the arms over the head, interlock the fingers and turn the palms upwards.
- Exhale and bend to the right side from the waist.
- Hold the position for a few seconds, breathing normally.
- Inhale and slowly come up to the upright position.
- Repeat the same on the left side. This would complete one round.
- Practise five to 10 rounds.

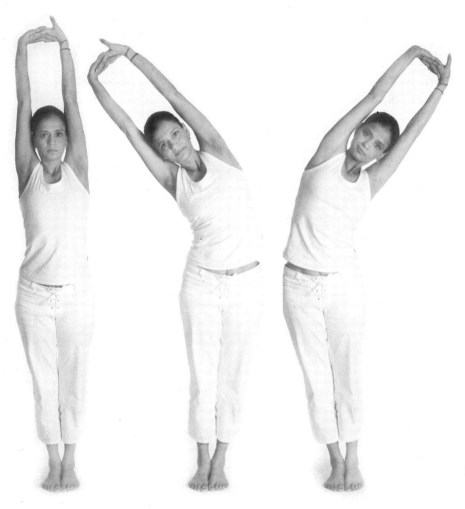

27

VIRKASANA (TREE POSE)

This posture strengthens the bone mass by increasing the weight pressure on the legs, hips and the spine and is helpful in osteoporosis. It improves balance and concentration, strengthens the muscles of the legs and the pelvis, opens the chest and shoulders and improves the quality of the breath.

- Stand with feet together, arms by the side and head straight.
- Bend the right leg at the knee and place the right heel firmly at the root of the left thigh, toes pointing downward.
- Balance on the left leg, join the palms and lowly raise the arms over the head.
- Focus the eyes on a stationary point on the wall and hold the posture for a few seconds, breathing normally.
- Release the posture by placing the right leg and arms down and repeat the same *asana* on the left side.
- Take care; practise the posture against the wall for support and balance.

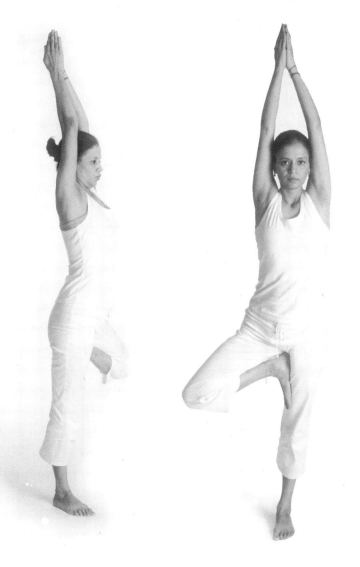

29

Vaksa-Sthala-Sakti Virasaka (Chest Expander Pose)

This *asana* increases the circulation to the upper half of the body, stretching the tense muscles in the upper body.

- Stand with feet hip-distance apart and head straight.
- Extend the arms behind the back and interlock the fingers.
- Expanding the chest, press the shoulders towards each other and breathe deeply. Stay in this position for 10 to 20 seconds.
- Inhale, contract the hip muscles and tighten the legs, bending backwards from the waist.
- Drop the head backwards and look upwards, releasing the stiffness from the shoulders and the neck.
- Stay in this position for a few seconds, breathing normally. Inhale and return to the start position.
- Exhale; bend forward from the waist, bringing the interlocked hands and arms up over the back.
- Relax the neck muscles and keep the knees straight. Hold for a few seconds, breathing normally.
- Inhale and return to the upright position.
- Repeat the entire sequence five to six times.
- Take care to interlock the hands as far as you can without feeling any discomfort.

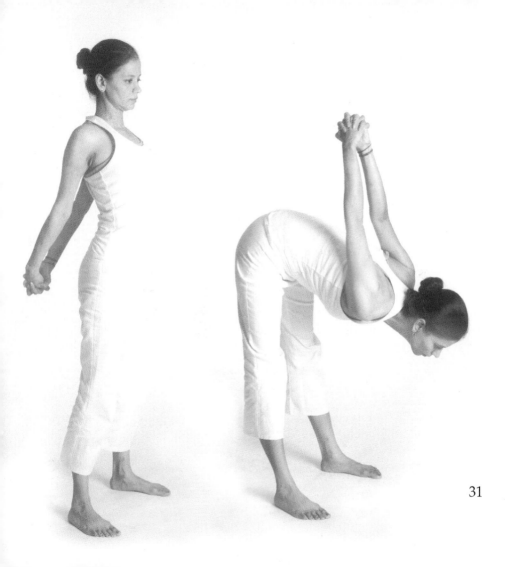

31

Janu-Sakti Vikasaka (**Bend Knee Pose**)

This *asana* tones the knees and is good for arthritic conditions of the knees as it improves the circulation of blood in the region. It also strengthens the calf muscles and the ankles besides toning the thighs.

- Stand with feet together, arms by the side.
- Bend the knees slightly and place both arms on the bent knees.
- Breathing normally, gently rotate the knees in a clockwise direction and complete 10 rounds.
- Repeat the same in an anti-clockwise direction for 10 rounds.
- Straighten the knees to release the posture.

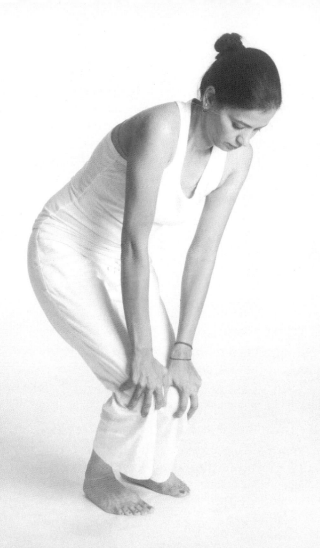

TRIKONASANA (TRIANGLE POSE)

This *asana* stretches the spine and the spinal nerves laterally and tones the entire body. It also increases the flexibility in the hips, stretches the back of the legs, strengthens the pelvic area and tones down the reproductive organs.

- Stand with feet together and arms by the side.
- Separate the legs 3 to 3.5 feet apart. Turn the right foot 90 degrees to the right and the left foot slightly by moving the heel away.
- Raise both the arms out to the sides and breathe in this position for a few seconds.
- Now lower the left arm and place the forearm on the lower back.
- Exhale. Bend towards the right and touch the right knee. Hold this position for a few seconds, breathing normally.
- Exhale and raise the left arm up towards the left and turn the head to look at the left hand.
- Hold this position for 10 to 20 seconds and slowly release the posture.
- Repeat the same on the left side.
- Take care not to over-stretch as the flexibility will improve with regular practice of this *asana*.

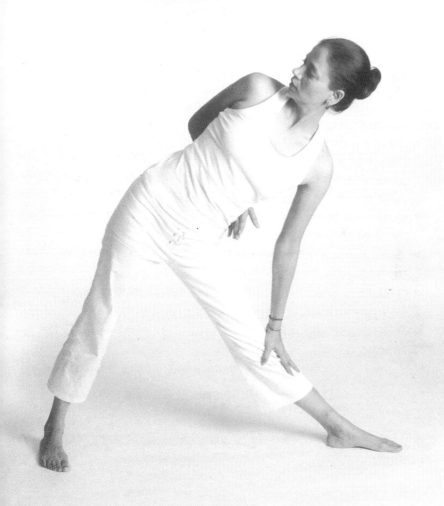

Supta Pavana Muktasana
(Half Wind-releasing Pose)

This _asana_ gives a wholesome effect to the entire body, besides toning the abdominal organs and helping in release of gas from the stomach. At the same time, it tones the thighs, knees and the toes.

- Lie flat on the floor with legs together and arms by the side.
- Raise the right leg and bend it from the knee. Hold it firmly against the chest by encircling it with the arms.
- Exhale; raise the head and shoulders up to touch the forehead to the right knee.
- Simultaneously raise the left leg 2 to 3 inches above the floor, flexing both the feet out.
- Hold the posture for 15 to 20 seconds, breathing normally.
- Exhale. Place the head and left leg down; raise the right leg and release the posture.
- Repeat the same with the left leg.

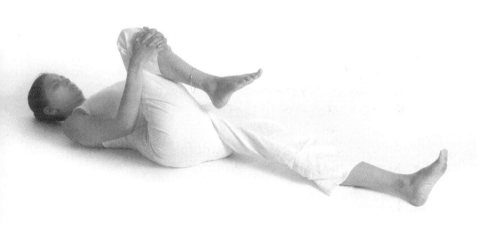

Uttan Padasana (Single Leg Lift)

These postures improve blood circulation throughout the pelvis and improve the working of the ovaries besides relieving menopausal symptoms, such as hot flashes and excessive bleeding in pre-menopausal women. At the same time, it strengthens the spine and the abdominal muscles. It is also helpful for varicose veins and improves circulation in the legs, improves concentration and relieves fatigue.

- Lie flat on the floor with legs together and arms by the side.
- Exhale, and raise the right leg up to a 90-degree angle. Keep the back flat on the floor and relax the entire body. Raise both arms up to hold the outer side of the right knee. Try to keep the knee straight.
- Hold the posture for as long as you feel comfortable, breathing normally.
- Release the posture by slowly lowering the arms and leg down.
- Repeat the same on the left side of the leg.
- Take care not to jerk the leg up and if you are unable to hold the knee, then hold on to the thighs or use a tie or a strap to hold the leg.

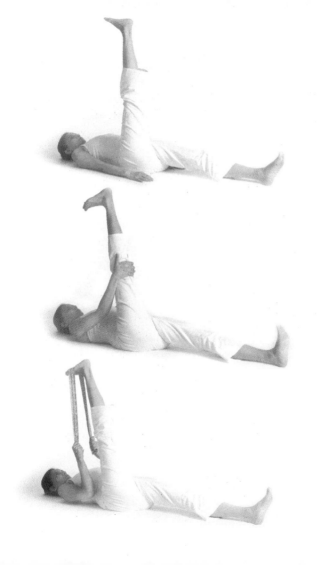

39

Supta Matsyendrasana (Reclining Twist)

This *asana* releases all the stiffness from the entire spine increasing its flexibility, improving digestion and toning all the organs of the abdomen.

- Lie flat on the floor with legs together and arms by the side.
- Turn on to your right side. Bend the left knee, place the left foot above or below the right knee, and let the bent knee rest on the floor.
- Extend both arms in front of you and gaze at the fingertips.
- Inhale. Lift the left arm upward in an arc by moving over and behind the body, ending with your arms in a T-position. Keeping the hips and legs towards the right, turn the head towards the left giving a twist to the spine.
- Hold this posture, breathing normally for 10 to 20 seconds.
- Release the posture, lift the left knee and straighten the leg and relax.
- Repeat the same on the other side.

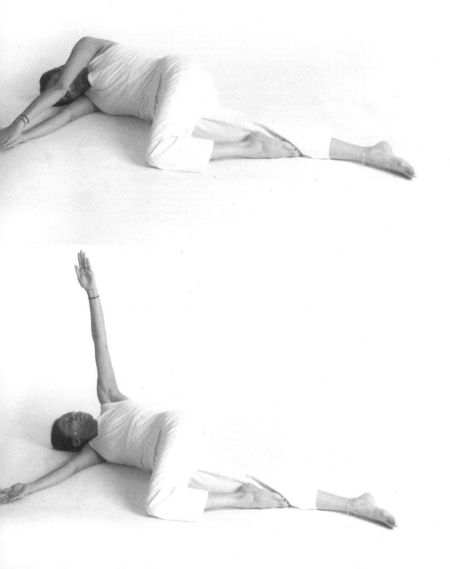

Supta Konasana (Wide Angle Pose)

- Lie on the back with legs against the wall and hips close to the wall, buttocks on the floor.
- Separate the legs and extend them out in a V with the arms extended to the side or under the neck.
- Breathe normally, holding this posture for 30 to 60 seconds and allowing the inner thighs to relax.
- Bring the legs together and hold this posture for 30 to 60 seconds.
- Exhale, lower the legs down and release the posture.
- Repeat this two to three times.
- Take care to spread the legs as far as comfortable. When you gain confidence, try and repeat this posture without the support of the wall.

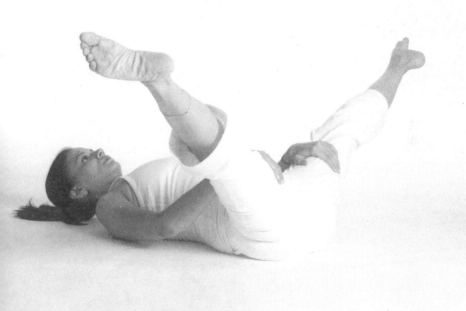

Ardh Chakrasana (Half Wheel)

This *asana* increases flexibility of the spine and is very helpful for balancing the hormones. At the same time it tones the legs, hips and the reproductive organs.

- Lie flat on the floor with legs a hip-distance apart and the arms by the sides with palms facing the floor.
- Bend the knees, keeping the feet flat and hold the ankles with both the hands.
- Inhale; raise the hips off the floor, arching the back upwards and raising the chest and navel as high as possible to touch the chin.
- Hold the posture, breathing normally for 2 to 30 seconds.
- Release the posture by resting the hips down and straighten the legs.

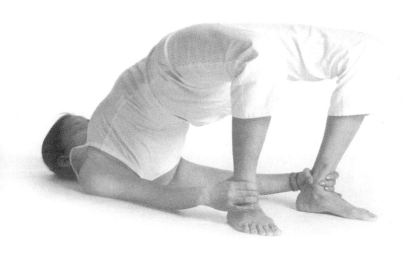

45

Viparita Karni (Inverted Pose)

This posture is a boon to women as it stimulates the thyroid gland and balances the circulatory, digestive, reproductive, nervous and endocrine systems. Since there is an enriched supply of blood to the brain, the mind becomes calm, gets rid of mental and emotional stress.

- Lie on the back with legs against the wall and hips close to the wall, buttocks on the floor.

OR

- Lie flat on the floor with legs together and arms by the side, close to the body, palms facing down.
- Pushing down on the arms and hands, raise both the legs up towards the head, rolling the lower back off the floor.
- Bend the elbows and turn the palms inward to support the lower back.
- Rest the hips on the palms and support the weight of the body on the elbows, neck and shoulders, keeping the trunk at a 45 degree angle from the floor, while maintaining the legs vertical.
- Breathe normally and hold the posture for as long as comfortable. Release the posture by bending the knees on the forehead and lower the spine on the floor.
- Take care to keep the spine well supported. Ensure that the knees do press against the chin. If you suffer from high blood pressure, avoid this posture.

46

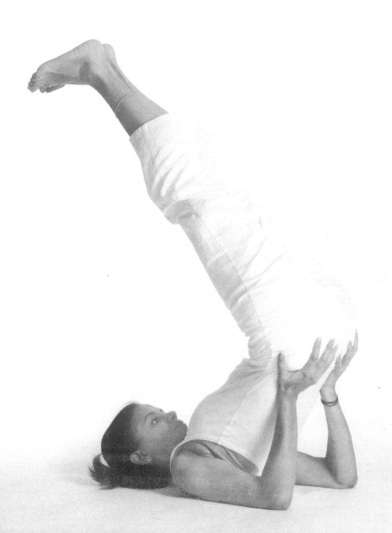

SARVANGASANA (SHOULDER STAND)

- Practice *Viparita Karni* for a few months and when you are confident, start the *Sarvangasana*. The benefits of this are the same as in the *Viparita Karni*.

- This *asana* is a straight continuation from *Viparita Karni.*

- Gently bring both the legs down at 40 degrees towards the forehead. Keep the back supported by the palms and gently push the spine straight with the support of the palms.

- Straighten the legs and bring them up to a vertical position, pressing the chin firmly into the base of your throat.

- Hold the posture for 30 seconds while breathing normally.

- Exhale, release the posture, lower the legs down and bend the knees on the forehead. Place the palms down and slowly roll down, breathing normally until the whole spine in resting on the floor.

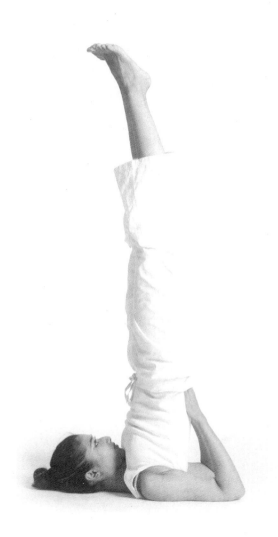

49

MATSYASANA (FISH POSE)

This *asana* helps the functioning of the thyroid gland and stimulates the thymus gland while boosting the immune system. It tones down the abdominal organs and since it stretches the chest, it is very useful in treating asthma and bronchitis. It tones the spine, neck and brings relief from throat ailments also.

- Lie flat on the floor with legs together and arms by the side.
- Inhale. Raise the head up, bend the elbows and rest the palms on the floor.
- Exhale; touch the head down on the floor, arching the back.
- Hold this posture for 20 to 30 seconds, breathing deeply.
- Inhale, lift the head up and place the head on the floor.

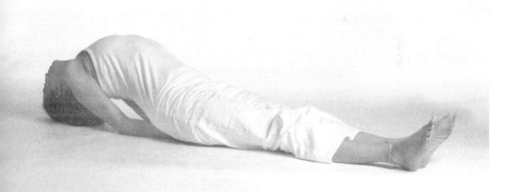

Ardh Shalabhasana (Half Locust Pose)

A series of these *asanas* energise the entire female reproductive organs and all the organs of the abdomen. These *asanas* are very helpful in women during their menopausal stage. This *asana* improves the circulation in the pelvic region, strengthens the lower back, legs and hips besides reducing the hot flashes through healthier ovarian function, lessening menopausal-related fatigue and improving the stamina and building your strength.

- Lie on the abdomen with legs together and arms by the side, close to the body.
- Slide the hands under the hips, palms facing the thighs. Lift the head up and extend forward to place the chin on the floor.
- Inhale. Keeping the left leg straight, lift the right leg as high as possible, using the back muscles.
- Exhale; lower the right leg down to its original place, and repeat this on the other side.
- Repeat this exercise 10 times with both the legs.
- Take care to keep the hips resting on the palms.

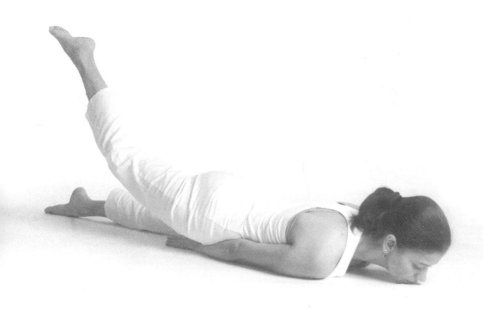

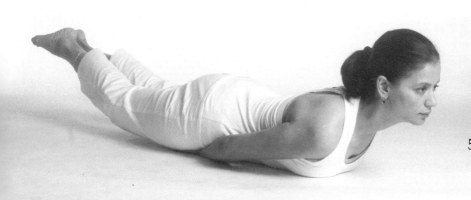

Ardh Bhujanasana (Sphinx Pose)

The regular practice of this posture removes backache and keeps the spine supple and healthy. It tones the ovaries and uterus, and alleviates gynaecological disorders.

- Lie on the abdomen with forehead touching the floor. Place the palms flat on the floor, just beyond the head, touching the thumb to the thumb and bending from the elbows.

- Inhale, contract the body below your navel and roll the head up, brushing the tip of the nose. Lift the chest off the floor, giving an elongating effect to the entire spine.

- Exhale; slowly lower the chest, chin and nose before finally touching the forehead on the floor.

- Repeat this three to four times.

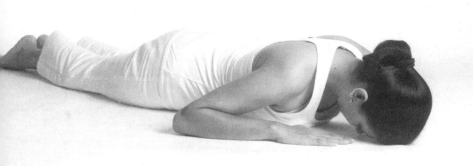

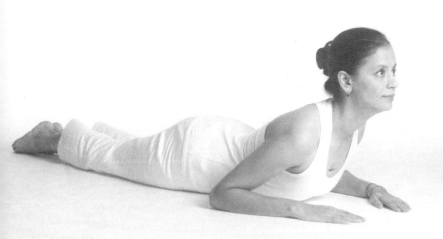

MAKARASANA (CROCODILE POSE)

This *asana* is excellent for women with lower back pain and spondilitis. It releases all the compression from the spinal nerves and at the same time proves helpful in lung ailments. It tones the toes, knees and the hips.

- Lie down on the abdomen with forehead touching the floor, arms close to the hips and ankles together.
- Raise the head and shoulders, bend and extend the elbows and rest the chin on the palms.
- Inhale, bend the legs from the knees and lift them up.
- Exhale, bring the legs down and begin again.
- Repeat five to 10 times.

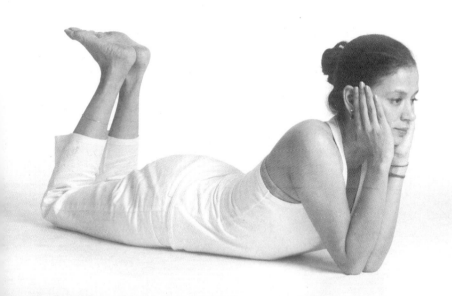

NAUKASANA (BOAT POSE)

This *asana* is excellent for women suffering from slip disc and sciatica pain. It tones the entire spine and the spinal nerves while at the same time toning the abdominal and reproductive organs. It also releases stiffness from the shoulders and tones the entire body.

- Lie on the abdomen with forehead touching the floor and arms close to the body.
- Lift the arms and extend them out in front with both palms joined together in *namaste* position.
- Exhale; lift the head, hands and your legs off the floor, balancing the body on the abdomen.
- Hold the posture, breathing normally for 10 to 20 seconds.
- Repeat the posture two to three times.
- Take care to contract the knees, the thighs and hips, while extending the shoulders out.

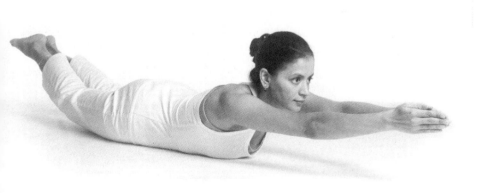

BIDALASANA (CAT POSE)

This pose relieves pain in the lower back and makes the spine flexible.

- Sit in the kneeling position.

- Place the hands on the floor, palms under the shoulders, fingers facing out and knees on the floor, with toes flexed out under the hips.

- Exhale. Bend the right knee and try to touch the knee to the nose or the forehead. Contract the abdominal muscles, tuck in the pelvis and arch the back upwards.

- Inhale, release the abdominal muscles, lift the right leg straight out as you lift yourself to the sitting posture. Spread the hips up, lifting the head and arching the spine down.

- Repeat this posture five to eight times on each side.

- Take care to keep the arms straight and the weight evenly distributed between the hands and the knees.

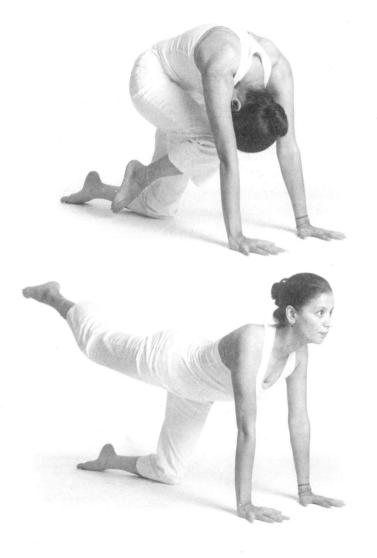

61

Ardh Dhanurasana (Half Bow)

This *asana* relieves all the stiffness in the spine and at the same time it is very beneficial for all respiratory problems, like asthma and bronchitis. It tones the shoulders and the hips.

- Lie down on the abdomen with forehead touching the floor, feet together and arms close to the body.
- Lift the arms up and extend out in front at shoulder-distance apart. With palms touching the floor, separate the legs hip-distance apart.
- Bend the right leg from the knee and touch the ankle on to the hips.
- Raise the right arm and reach out to hold the right ankle.
- Inhale, raise the right leg off the floor, arching the spine. Simultaneously lift the left arm, head and chest.
- Hold the posture, breathing normally for 10 to 20 seconds.
- Exhale, lower the body and the right leg on the floor.
- Repeat the same on the other side.

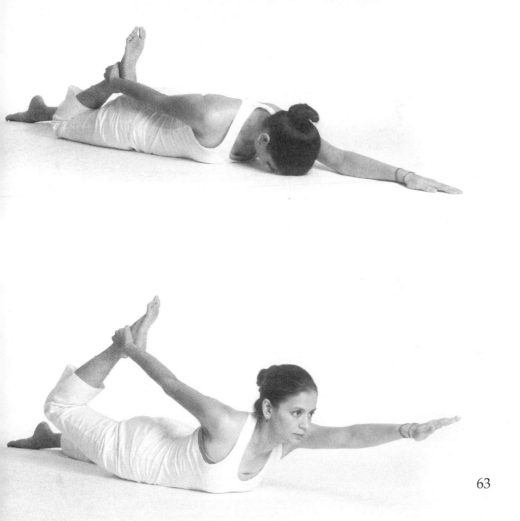

Baddhakon Asana (Butterfly Pose)

This *asana* increases the flexibility of the hips, inner thighs, pelvis, lower back, knees and the ankles. It tones the reproductive organs and is also very helpful in correcting menstrual problems.

- Sit on the floor with the spine held straight.
- Bend your knees; join the soles of your feet together by bringing your heels inward to your pelvis.
- Hold your feet with hands and press your knees downward to the floor. If you cannot hold this pose, flap your knees up and down gently instead.
- Lift your lower back and elongate by extending your entire spine for 20 to 30 seconds.
- Then bend forward from the hips.
- Place your elbows on your inner thighs and keep pressing down, at the same time extending your torso towards the floor.
- Rest your forehead on the ground.
- To release the posture, gently lift the head up and relax.

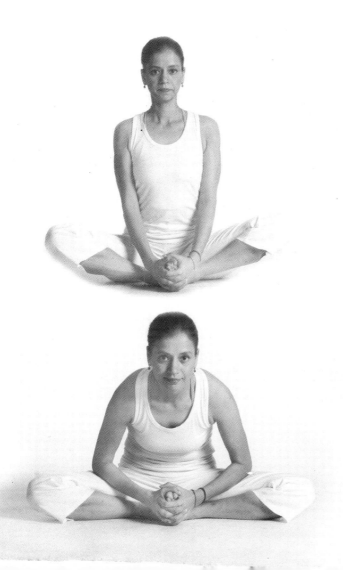

65

Paschimottan Asana (SEATED FORWARD BEND)

This *asana* rejuvenates the entire spine and the abdomen, toning the internal organs. It also helps in removing skin pigmentation that occurs due to hormonal changes in menopausal women.

It soothes and calms the mind and the nervous system; it tones the abdominal muscles, the uterus and the ovaries while enhancing their functions.

- Sit on the floor with legs together and stretched out in front. Place your palms on the floor by the side of your hips and keep the spine erect.
- Inhale; raise both arms straight up, stretching the spine upwards.
- Exhale, and bend forward to reach out for your toes, or ankles or the shin bone. If possible, touch your forehead on the knees.
- Hold the posture for 10 to 20 seconds, breathing normally.
- Inhale, and lift yourself back into the starting position.
- Repeat the posture two to three times.
- Take care to keep the knees and back straight or support the spine and the knees with cushions as shown in the picture.

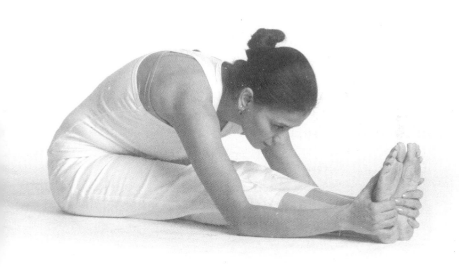

67

MARICHYASANA (SPINAL TWIST)

This posture rejuvenates the entire spinal nerves and makes the back flexible. It tones all the abdominal organs, regulates the secretion of the adrenaline and bile and is extremely helpful in curing diabetes, pre-menopausal bleeding, urinary tract infection and spondylitis.

- Sit on the floor with legs together and stretched out in front. Place your palms on the floor by the side of your hips and keep the spine erect.
- Place the left leg straight and the right leg crossed over the left leg, near the left knee.
- Raise your right arm up and take it behind to place it behind the back. Keep the palm on the floor and with fingers pointing away from the hips, lift the left arm and wrap it around the right knee, hugging the knee to the chest before looking over the right shoulder.
- Hold the posture for 10 to 20 seconds, breathing normally.
- Take care to keep the neck in a neutral position if you feel any strain or stretching on the neck.

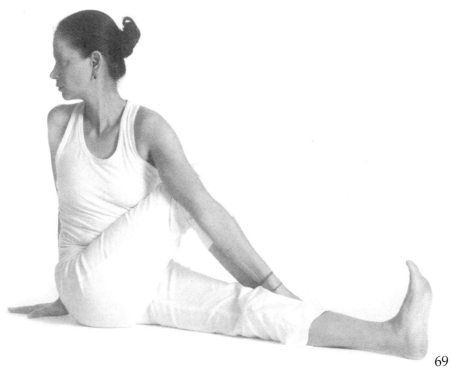

69

SIMHASANA (LION POSE)

This *asana* tones the back, knees and at the same time helps in reducing wrinkles, toning the eye muscles and helping in oral treatment. It clears the throat and makes the voice clearer. It improves memory and concentration too.

- Sit on your shins with the hips on the heels.
- Keeping the toes together, separate the knees out one to two feet apart. Place the arms on the knees, palms facing the knees, and the spine straight.
- Inhale deeply, straightening the back.
- Exhale loudly through the mouth, taking your tongue out and pressing it on the chin. Focus the eyes on the tip of the nose.
- Hold this position, breathing normally.
- Inhale, pull the tongue in, and relax the eyes.
- Repeat the posture two to four times.

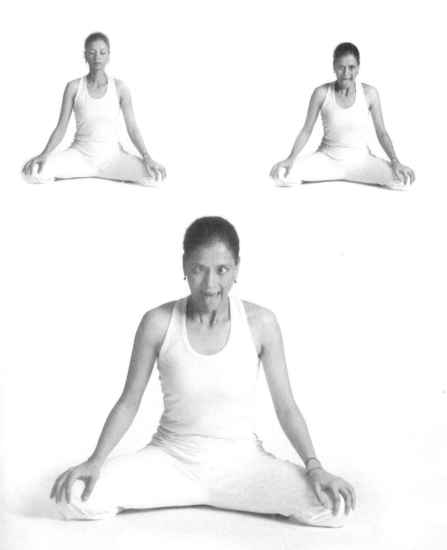

Salamba Bharadvajasana (Supported Twist)

This *asana* is excellent for soothing the tired nerves and is a must for women as it gently stretches the back muscles. It relaxes the mind and body and thus fosters their health.

- Sit on your shins with your hips on the heels.
- Place a stack of folded blankets near the right ankle and keep it pointing away from you.
- Exhale, move the spine to the right and place your hands on the floor on either side of the blankets. Then slowly lower the torso on to the blankets and lower your head on it.
- Let the left thigh rise away from the heels and your right hip will slip down between the right ankle and the edge of the blankets.
- Let the legs separate slightly and release them towards the floor.
- Hold this posture for one to two minutes, breathing normally and relaxing the entire body.
- Inhale, lift yourself up and repeat the same on the other side.
- Take care to adjust the height of the blankets so that you can settle in a comfortable position.

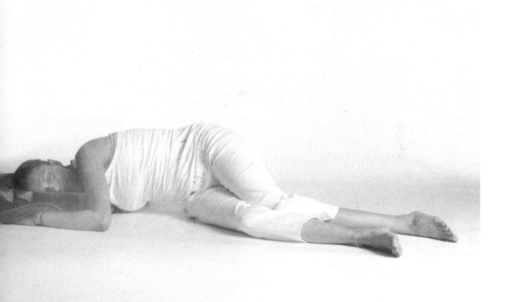

73

Savasana (Corpose Pose)

This posture releases all the fatigue from the body and the stress from the mind. It relaxes the entire nervous system and recharges the body and mind.

- Lie flat on your back, on the floor. Keep the arms stretched out alongside your body with palms facing downwards.
- Separate the legs 2 cms apart, keeping the toes relaxed and feet lying naturally.
- Separate the arms 5 inches away from the body, palms facing upward and fingers naturally relaxed.
- Close your eyes and shift the awareness on breathing and shut out all external sounds.
- Stay in this posture for 10 minutes.
- Gently bring some awareness in the body and roll your neck from side to side; then roll to the right and raise the body up.

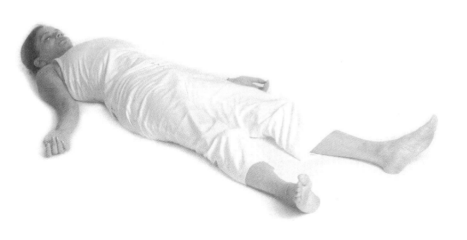

75

8

Pranayama

The process of breathing occurs in our body automatically, spontaneously and naturally. We are breathing even when we are not aware of it because breathing is important for the body for two reasons. It is the only means to supply our bodies and its organs with a good supply of oxygen, and is very vital for our survival and secondly, it gets rid of all the toxins from the body. Most people do not know the correct way of breathing and this results in using only a small part of your lung capacity. This type of 'shallow breathing' actually deprives your body of the right quantity of oxygen essentially required for your body's health and results in toxic buildup. Our resistance to disease is reduced, since oxygen is essential for healthy cells.

Yogis have studied the process of breathing in detail and have come to know that there exists a strong connection between breathing and the state of mind and they have developed a scientific method to control this process which they call *pranayama*. This is made up off two Sanskrit words, *prana* means 'life-force' and *yama* meaning 'to control'. *Pranayama* is a *yogic* science of breathing and regulating this vital energy (*prana*) in our system by controlling the breath. *Pranayama* consists of a series of breathing exercises, especially intended to bring a perfect balance in the body and mind and help keep the body vibrant and healthy. In *pranayama* we focus our attention on the breath and when we follow the breath, the mind is also drawn into the activities of the breath, thus preparing you for the stillness of meditation. While we discuss *pranayama* we must clearly understand three technical terms related to it and these are *puraka*, *rechaka* and *kumbhaka*.

Puraka (inhalation) should be slow, deep and complete with no extra force applied for taking in air. The lungs should be filled completely with air and it should be uniform.

Rechaka (exhalation) should be controlled, slow, deep and uniform. The lungs should be emptied to the maximum extent.

Kumbhaka (retention) involves stopping of all movements of breath by holding the entire respiratory apparatus still.

There is a fixed proportion of time to be maintained regarding these three and it is recommended that *rechaka* (exhalation) should be double the time of *puraka* (exhalation) and the *kumbhaka* (retention) depends upon the progress of each individual practice.

Regular practice of *pranayama* will help release all the pre- and post-menopausal symptoms like hot flashes, stress, anxiety and hormonal imbalances. There will be a tremendous improvement in the health of the nervous system, including the brain, spinal cord, nerves centres, thus improving the health of the entire body. *Yogic* breathing reduces the workload on the heart and results in a healthy and a strong heart. The process of slow deep breathing results in release of all toxins from the body and rejuvenating of the skin. This helps in reduction of facial wrinkles. Practice of *pranayama* relaxes the mind and the body as the slow, deep, rhythmic breathing causes a reflex stimulation of the parasympathetic nervous system, which results in reduction in the heart rate and relaxation of the muscles. Above all, *pranayama* helps you to connect spiritually which is very important at this phase of life.

So let us begin the journey of a healthy relationship between the mind and the body through the regular practice of *pranayama*.

SEETKARI (TEETH HISSING)

Pranayama cools the entire body and has an excellent relaxing effect upon the whole body. It is very helpful in reducing the hot flashes that women experience during menopause. It also induces mental and emotional stability and a feeling of tranquillity.

- Sit in a comfortable cross-legged position with hands on the thighs, palms facing up and the thumb touching the index finger (*chin mudra*).
- Hold the back straight, shoulders relaxed and chin parallel to the floor.
- Close your eyes and relax the body while doing mind breathing, normally for a few seconds.
- Touch the tongue to the palate, clench your teeth together and keep the lips slightly open.
- Inhale, slowly and deeply, through the teeth and at the end of the inhalation close the lips.
- Exhale slowly and deeply from the nostrils.
- This completes one round.
- Repeat five to 10 rounds.

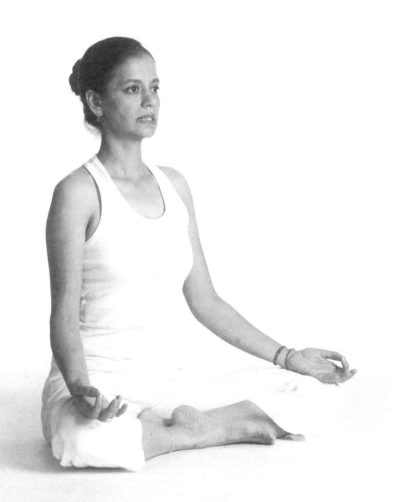

81

Anuloma Viloma (Alternate Nostril Breathing)

The regular practice of this *pranayama* will balance the entire nervous system and calm the mind, clear all the blockages in the nasal passages and cure one from all diseases.

- Sit in a comfortable cross-legged position with the back straight and hand on the palms.
- The left hand is kept in *chin mudra,* the thumb touching the index finger and with the right hand in Vishnu *mudra,* tuck your index and middle finger.
- Inhale through the left nostril, closing the right nostril with the thumb, to the count of 4.
- Hold the breath, closing both nostrils to the count of 16.
- Exhale through the right nostril, closing the left nostril with the ring and the little finger, to the count of 8.
- Inhale through the right nostril, keeping the left nostril closed with the ring finger and little finger, to the count of 4.
- Hold the breath to the count of 16.
- Exhale through the left nostril, keeping the right nostril closed with the thumb to the count of 8.
- This completes one round of alternate nostril breathing. Begin with four rounds and gradually build up to 20 rounds.

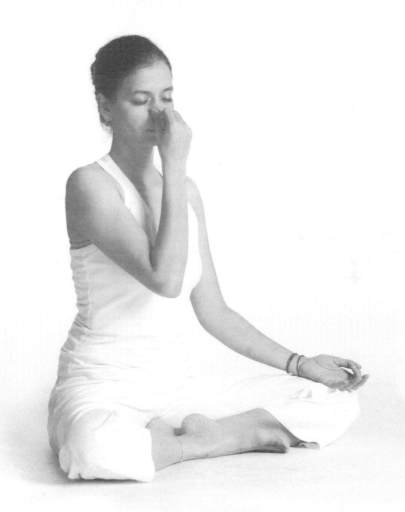

Bhramari Pranayama (**Humming Bee**)

This *pranayama* relieves stress and tension, alleviates mood swings, reduces blood pressure and insomnia. It harmonises the mind and directs the awareness inward.

- Sit in a comfortable cross-legged position with hands on the thigh and palms facing upward.
- Close the eyes and relax the whole body by breathing deeply.
- Raise the arms and bend the elbows, bringing the hands to the ears. Use the index finger to plug the ear.
- Inhale, slowly and deeply.
- Exhale, slowly making a deep, smooth and steady humming sound like that of the bee.
- This completes one round.
- Practise five to 10 rounds.

9

Bandha

Bandha are the locks that have a powerful effect on the flow of *prana* and they also have a powerful effect on the reproductive organs of the women. They tone the internal muscles of the body and at the same time divert the energy towards calming and stilling the mind to connect you spiritually. They help in altering the mood swings and enhance awareness and concentration.

Moolabandha (Anal Lock)

Regular practice of this *bandha* tones the perineal area and pelvic floor muscles; it increases blood flow to the pelvic region, encouraging the maintenance of healthy vaginal and urethral tissues.

- Sit in a comfortable cross-legged position, hands on the thighs and the palms touching the knees.
- Keep the spine straight.
- Close your eyes and relax the body by breathing deeply.
- Inhale slowly and deeply, contracting the sphincter and vaginal muscles as if trying to hold back urination. Contract the perinal and pelvic floor muscles.
- Hold the contraction for a few breaths.
- Exhale; release the contraction to begin again.

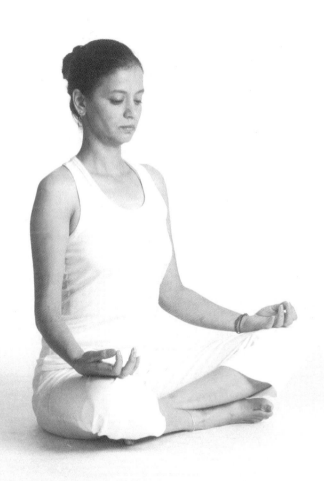

Uddiyana Bandha (Abdominal Lock)

The practice of this *bandha* stimulates the digestive process as all the abdominal organs are toned and massaged. It also improves the blood circulation and strengthens the reproductive organs. Thus it proves a boon for women in menopause.

- Sit in a comfortable cross-legged position with the spine straight, the knees touching the floor and the palms on the knees.
- Close the eyes and relax the entire body by breathing deeply.
- Inhale slowly and deeply.
- Exhale all the air from the lungs, drawing your navel and abdomen inward into your thoracic cavity, toward the spine.
- Retain the breath for a few seconds without straining.
- Release the lock by inhaling slowly and deeply and then resume normal breathing.
- Practise two to three times.

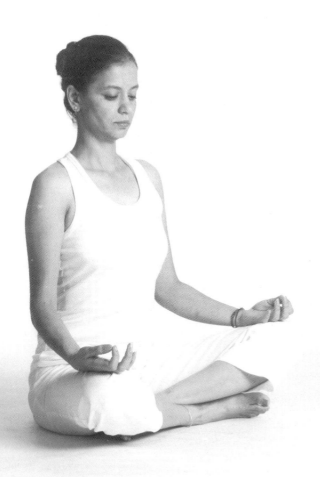

89

JALANDHARA BANDHA OR CHIN LOCK

This practice regulates your respiratory and circulatory systems, relieves stress and anxiety, producing a state of mental relaxation. The pressing of your chin to your throat helps to balance your thyroid function and to regulate the metabolism.

- Sit in a comfortable cross-legged position with the spine erect and palms placed on your knees. Close your eyes and relax your body.

- Inhale slowly and deeply. Retain your breath and as you do so, drop your head forward and press your chin tightly against your chest.

- Stay in this position for as long as you can, holding your breath without any strain.

- Release the chin lock, raise your head and exhale.

- Practise three rounds of this posture.

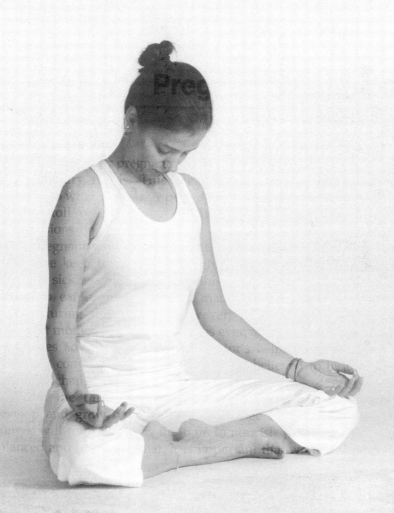

10

Mudras

M*udras* are defined as gestures that have a powerful effect on the attitude of the *prana* flow. They help in altering the mood, the attitude and to deepen one's awareness and attitude. Each *mudra* has a subtle effect on the mind as it moves inward and one can experience a sense of withdrawal.

Hridaya Mudra (Heart Seal)

This *mudra* has a profound effect on the heart area, as the *prana* flows from the hands to the heart area, improving the condition of the heart. It is helpful in finding release from all emotions and calms the heart.

- Sit in a comfortable cross-legged position with the spine held straight and knees touching the floor.
- Place the index fingers at the root of the thumb, and join the tips of the middle and ring fingers to the tips of the thumbs, with the little fingers kept straight.
- Place the hand on the knees with palms facing upward.
- Close the eyes and relax the body by shifting the awareness on the breath and keeping the body still.
- Stay in this position for as long as you feel comfortable.

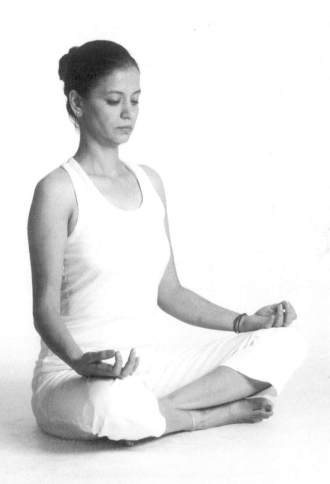

95

Ajna Mudra (Internal Eye Seal)

This *mudra* strengthens the eye muscles and releases tension in this area. It will mentally calm you down and prepare you for meditation. It also activates the pineal glands and balances all the emotions.

- Sit in a comfortable cross-legged position with knees touching the floor and palms on the knees in *chin mudra*.

- Close the eyes, and relax the body by breathing deeply for a few seconds.

- Open the eyes and slowly focus the eyes at the centre of eyebrows for 10 seconds; then close the eyes.

- Next, repeat the same but with eyes closed for 10 seconds.

- Hold this for as long as possible, breathing normally and meditating on the stillness.

- Take care to open the eyes at the slightest tension or strain.

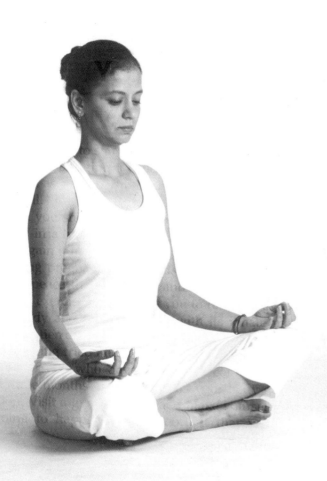

97

11

Kriya

The *kriyas* are techniques that help in purification of the body of all toxins. According to *hatha* yoga, the body needs to be totally clean and only then can the benefits of *asanas* and *pranayama* be felt. The main aim of these *kriyas* is to create harmony between the right and the left nostrils by bringing about physical and mental purification and balance and helping to clean the eyes.

KAPALBHATI (PURIFICATION OF NOSTRILS)

In Sanskrit, *kapala* means the 'skull' and *bhati* means 'shining'. As a one word, *kapalbhati* means that if you practise this *pranayama*, your face will glow with good health. This *pranayama* purifies your entire system and releases toxins from your body. Your mind gets energised and prepared for meditation. It strengthens your nervous system and tones your digestive organs.

- Sit in a comfortable crossed-legged position, keeping your spine straight and hands resting on your knees in the *chin mudra*. Relax your body and breathe deeply.

- Inhale deeply through the nostrils, expanding your abdomen.

- Exhale with a forceful contraction of your abdominal muscles, expelling the air out of your lungs.

- Inhale again but passively allow your abdominal muscles to expand and inflate your lungs with air without any force. This is going to be a pumping effect of passive inhalation and expulsion of breath in a continuous manner.

- Do eight or 10 breath expulsions. Then inhale and exhale deeply for two rounds followed by retaining of breath for 20 to 30 seconds.

- Practise three rounds of *kapalbhati*.

- Take care not to strain while performing this *pranayama*. Your facial muscles should be relaxed. If you feel any pain or dizziness, stop the practice for some time. Those who suffer from high blood pressure, vertigo, any ear or eye complaint, they should avoid this posture.

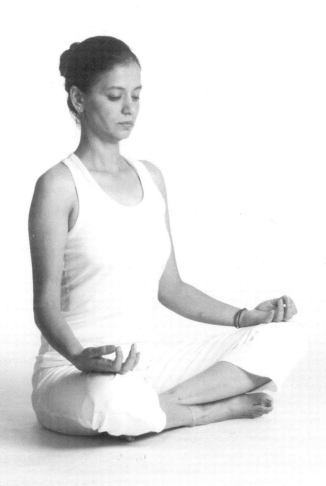

Tratka (Purification of Eyes)

The practice of this *kriya* removes all the defects of eyesight, releases all nervous tension, anxiety, depression, improves memory and develops a strong will power. It is of particular benefit in developing spiritual powers.

- Light a candle and place it on a small table so that the flame is exactly at eye level when sitting and the candle is kept arms-length away from the body.

- Sit in a comfortable cross-legged position, knees touching the floor, hands on the knees and palms in *chin mudra* or else sit on your shins.

- Close your eyes and relax the body for a few minutes, keeping the body totally still.

- Open your eyes and gaze steadily at the wick of the candle and try not to blink. When the eyes become tired or begin to water, close the eyes.

- Close your eyes and focus at the point between the eyebrows and visualise the image of the flame in the space in front of the closed eyes, till the image begins to fade.

- Open the eyes and begin again.

- Repeat this three to five times.

- After you finish the rounds, rub both palms together, make a cup of the palms and gently place them over your eyes.

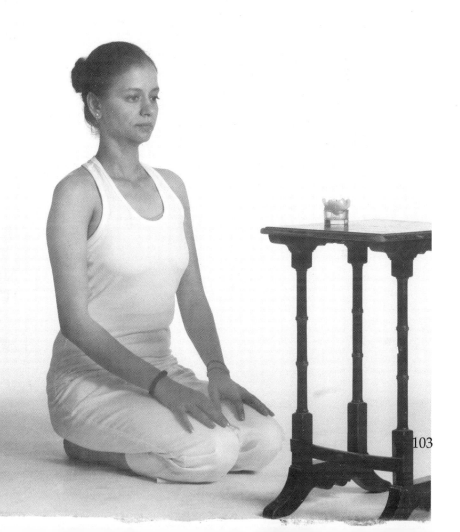

103

12

Meditation

Meditation is the practice of freeing the mind of all the worries and pains that surround us. To achieve this total state of happiness and to free ourselves, we must meditate regularly; this will teach us to explore our inner dimension. Meditation is not a ritual and does not belong to any particular culture; it belongs to all and through this we can find the eternal truth. It is the process of stilling the mind against outside distractions to discover peace and wisdom within yourself. Regular meditation will make you acquire a greater sense of who you are and what you are looking for in your life. Above all, it helps you to concentrate your mind and calmly face external influences.

At this point of life when women are experiencing physical as well as mental stress, it becomes necessary to meditate and release emotional stress from the body and mind. Meditation will help you cope with this new life and understand that this is a natural process of life which every woman must experience and meditation will help you understand it better. Meditation is therapeutic as it cures the body of various ailments like blood pressure and reduces the possibilities of heart attack. It also helps in curing diabetes and works like a tonic for the body. Meditation brings in calmness with peace and release of energy. The focus of all meditation practice is to control the busy mind. What is needed is concentration of the mind on one healing element—one sound, one image or one breath. This will bring in inner peace and calmness and the mind will not take off on its own thoughts of worry and get stressed and depressed.

So let's begin the journey with a few points to remember.

- Find a simple quiet place where no one can distract you. Establish a suitable time for your practice and do the practice every day at the same time.

- Choose a suitable posture in which you can sit comfortably for more than half an hour. Work on stilling the body by sitting in this posture and relax the body.

- Bring awareness on the breath or on whatever object you choose and stick to it.

- Be patient and keep up your practice.

- To keep your balance throughout the posture is very important. Take time out to practice the simple techniques of meditation as these will lead to inner balance and stability and help to cure you of inner complexes.

MITTA MEDITATION

This meditation has a calming effect. As all thoughts are released from your mind, you will feel a state of immense silence and stillness. Develop an attitude of love towards yourself.

- Sit in a meditative posture. Relax your body and breathe.
- Focus on that part of your breath that is touching the sides of your nostrils. Let the thoughts come and go without distracting you.
- Inhale. Let your breath flow at its natural pace, but focus on chanting in your mind, the following, 'May I be peaceful and joyful, may my body be well.'
- Continue to do this for at least 20 minutes and then lie down in *shavasana*.

JOURNEY MEDITATION

This meditation involves visualisation and appeals to women who desire to picturise themselves in a peaceful place. It is also an excellent way to improve the full mood for the day and proves helpful when you are at the lowest energy level.

- Sit in a comfortable cross-legged position or on a low stool.
- Relax the body and breathe by taking breaths deeply and slowly.
- Relax the facial muscles and close the eyelids.
- Become aware of all the problems, concerns and fears, telling the mind that you will take care of them once you are through with your meditation.
- Now breathe in slowly and deeply for 4 counts and exhale for 8 counts for a few seconds.
- Take your mind to a peaceful place, where you feel serene, safe and calm. A quiet walk in the mountains is an ideal place for many, or a beach for a few. Picture yourself resting on the sand on the shores of the calm sea or on the mountain slopes. Feel the sun on your skin; hear the water lapping the shore, listen to the chirping of the birds. Use the same routine at any peaceful place that calms you.

BREATH AND NAVEL MEDITATION

This meditation works directly with the natural flow of breath in the nostrils and with every expansion and contraction of the abdomen. This mediation is a good way to focus attention and inculcate pointed awareness.

- Sit in a comfortable cross-legged position or in a meditative position or in *shavasana* with palms on the abdomen.

- Relax the body and breathe deeply and slowly.

- Press the tongue to the palate, close the mouth without clenching the teeth and close the eyelids.

- Breathe naturally through the nostrils. Focus on the gentle breeze of air flowing in and out of the nostrils and on the navel rising and falling with the entire abdomen expanding and contracting like a balloon at every inhalation and exhalation.

- Whenever you catch the mind wandering off or getting cluttered with thoughts, shift your attention back to your breath.

13

Relaxation

Relaxation is defined as an activity that produces relief and diversion from work for the body and mind. It is a process to slow down and respond to all the challenges that one faces in life with greater equainimity. Relaxation techniques used in yoga are extremely simple and yet very beneficial as to produce a relaxed body and a joyful, clear mind.

It is an important part of yoga that each *hatha* yoga class must end with a 10 minutes of cooling down period. This is the *yogic* relaxation technique which is a guided relaxation and serves as a 'feel good' factor after a complete stretch.

Relaxation helps in release of stress from the body and calms the heart and the entire cardiovascular system, besides relaxing all the muscles and the entire nervous system.

It is very important to add this technique in your daily yoga practice. Yoga relaxation techniques help to calm your mind and you will experience a sense of inner peace and tranquillity. As you learn to handle all stresses in every phase of life, daily relaxation exercises will take away all your tension and fatigue and keep your body and mind rejuvenated.

Yoga *Nidra* (Systematic Relaxation)

- Lie down in *shavasana* (corpse pose).
- Breathe slowly and deeply for a few minutes, bringing awareness to the entire body.
- Now shift the awareness to the crown of the head and systematically move downwards, mentally scanning the entire body and relaxing each and every body part.
- Breathe as if the entire body is breathing and relax the entire body.
- Shift the awareness to the mind and release all thoughts from the mind. Even if a thought comes, just let it come and pass by, filling the mind with your breath.
- Relax yourself physically and mentally, staying in this position for as long as you want.
- Get some awareness back into the body, turn to the right and sit up in the meditative posture to continue with meditation for a few minutes more.
- Allow this posture to end on its own, as your body knows when it has benefited sufficiently and naturally to take you out of relaxation.

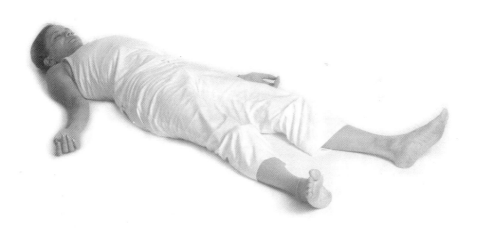

113

14

Eating Right Food

To get the most out of yoga, it is very important that you eat right. Food is our body's main source of energy and has a lot of healing and curative value. It has been rightly proved by *yogis* that our body and mind are made up of the food we eat. The first important rule here is to make healthy food choices.

In yogic terms, you need to eat *sattvic* food — pure and natural, that will increase your vigour and vitality and bring energy to your body. You should avoid *rajasic* (hot, bitter and dry) and *tamasic* food that is tasteless, impure, stale or rotten.

At this age the food we eat is extremely important, as a nutritious and balanced diet will help you overcome all medical problems associated with age.

In menopause, decreased hormone levels can contribute to deficiency of vitamins and minerals in the body with the result that the body can no longer maintain the calcium levels and there is loss of minerals from the bones. These symptoms are associated with osteoporosis. Eating a well-balanced diet can help you manage your symptoms and protect your bones and heart. Switch to natural and fresh foods for your nutritive requirements and these are available in abundance. Make sure the food eaten is as far as possible in its natural state or cooked very lightly as prolonged contact with heat destroys the food's nutritive value.

- Eat two to three servings of fruits daily. Drink lots of fruit juices as they supply the body with life-giving vitamins, minerals and fibre. Vegetables are as important as fruits and should preferably be cooked very lightly or eaten raw in the form of salads.

- Limit the number of calories in your diet that come from fat; no more than 30 per cent of your total calories can come from fat each day.

- Choose foods that are rich in calcium to make sure you get at least 1,500 mg of calcium per day. Milk and milk products, nuts, and dark green vegetables are high in calcium. If you think you are not getting enough calcium from your diet, talk to your doctor about taking a calcium supplement.

- Make sure your diet contains enough of proteins. Foods rich in protein are nuts, pulses, seeds, eggs, lentils, milk and cottage cheese.

- Include a good source of fibre in your diet, such as wheat grains, beans and corn every day.

- Start to take two servings of soya, the wonder food that has been proved to reduce menopausal symptoms.

- Maintain a healthy body weight.

Water is vital. It makes up two-thirds of the body weight and helps in flushing toxins out. Drink at least 10 to 12 glasses of water a day. Avoid drinking water half an hour before or after a meal, as it dilutes your gastric juices and hinders digestion

Vitamin A: Necessary for normal bone remodelling. In women with vitamin A deficiency, new bone forms faster than the old bone and abnormal bone formation occurs. Right intake of vitamin A promotes good eyesight, healthy skin and good teeth. Foods rich in vitamin A are milk and milk products, fruits and vegetables and eggs.

Vitamin B6: This vitamin is necessary for the absorption of useful minerals from dietary calcium sources. It aids in assimilation of fats and proteins and is essential for proper functioning of the nervous system. Foods rich in this vitamin are wheat germ, bran, brewer's yeast, milk, banana, peanuts, raisins, and cabbage.

Vitamin C: This vitamin promotes the formation of collagen, which aids in the synthesis of structural proteins found in the bone. It holds the body cells together and increases resistance to infection. Important sources of this vitamin are citrus fruits, leafy green vegetables and potatoes.

Vitamin D: Even a slight decrease in this vitamin leads to osteoporosis. Vitamin D enhances the uptake of calcium in the intestines, thereby allowing more calcium to be available for deposition in the bones. Women during menopause should ensure that their vitamin D intake is adequate; hence take eggs, fortified milk and expose yourself to ultraviolet rays of the sun

Vitamin K: Required for normal bone metabolism, this vitamin helps in maintenance of the blood-clotting system. This vitamin is found in green leafy vegetables and wheat grains.

Vitamin E: This vitamin works as an anti-oxidant and helps in the prevention of unwanted blood clots. It promotes better circulation and formation of new skin on wounds. It works very well along with vitamin C and helps in anti-ageing. All wheat grain products, wheat gram, green leafy vegetables, and vegetable oil contain vitamin E.

Here are some practical guidelines that will help you regulate your eating habits:

- Never ever overeat. This is the worst thing you can do to your body. Eat the right amount of food and according to your body's requirements and the physical activity you perform. Always remember to keep your stomach a little empty for your body to perform its natural function of digestion properly.

- Eat three meals a day or space your eating into four to five meals based on your body's needs. But make sure the quantity always remains the same.

- Never miss a breakfast, as it is the most important meal of the day after a fast of 10 to 12 hours. Breakfast gives you energy for the entire day.

- Make a deadline for the last meal of the day and ensure that you do not eat anything past this deadline.

- Replace the use of refined sugar with a healthier, natural sweetener like honey. Avoid food rich in spices as it leads to acidity and heartburn.

- Eat only freshly cooked food and not stale or old food that is kept in the fridge. Avoid deep fried food as it is indigestible and the nutrients are destroyed while frying.
- Fast at least once a month or go on a fruit juice diet. This is good as your body gets the time to put all the energy in and flush the toxins from the body.
- Try to cut down on the three whites from your diet—flour, sugar and salt.
- Avoid excess fat but a little is required to maintain lubrication of the joints.
- Maintain a diary to write your daily diet and exercise routine. Also note any deviations. Documentation will help you to stay focused, keep a track on any lapses and help you understand yourself better.

There is no doubt that with a proper diet and *yogic* discipline you will be able to cope better with this phase in your life. Remember to remain motivated and committed to your purpose.

15

Yogic Self-therapeutic Massage

Massage is derived from the Greek word *massier*, meaning 'to knead.' Massage is an excellent passive form of exercise and involves gentle pressing of the soft tissues of the body. Massaging is very therapeutic as it induces relaxation, reduces pain and stiffness in the body, and at the same time balances the overall energy flow in the body. Massage works directly on the muscles by use of different strokes for manipulation of the body. Regular messaging tones up the nervous system, influences respiration, eliminates toxins from the body, removes facial wrinkles, helps to curb depression, induces sleep and cures insomnia. Pamper yourself by a regular massage as it is therapeutic and provides relaxation and reduces emotional tension. If you don't have the time to go to the spa for a regular massage, you can do the spa treatment on your own at home, but keep in mind a few things before starting.

The first step in massage is choosing the oil depending on the body type—sesame oil is best for cool, dry skin as it warms and soothes the body. Coconut oil has a cooling effect and is suited to oily skin. There are five modes of manipulation in massage and these are:

Effleurage: This involves stroking and sliding the hands over the surface of the body so as to increase blood circulation and soothe the nervous system.

Petrissage: This process involves kneading, pressing and rolling of the soft tissues. This massage strengthens the muscles and helps in elimination of toxins from the body.

Friction: The movements are circular in nature and useful in breaking up the toxin deposits in the joints.

Tapotament: This involves tapping, clapping and beating the body rapidly in short and quick blows generally given from the wrists. It increases the blood supply, soothes the nerves and strengthens the muscles.

Vibration: This is achieved by shaking and pressing the fingers or hands on the body. It stimulates circulation and glandular activity.

A special massage done on the head and the neck is known as *shiro abhanga*. This massage focuses on the three energy points. The *Brahma Randhra* massage (the crown of the head) reduces headaches. *Adhipati* massage on top of the head and midway between the ears, reduces hypertension. *Manya mula* massage on the deep indentation at the base of the skull bone, just above the hairline on the back of the neck, treats pancreatic dysfunction. The head and neck massage should be done once a week with almond oil.

The next step in self-massage is to add an extra dimension of pleasure and healing by adding aromatherapy oil in the essential oil to blend the two and create an oil blend that calms and relaxes the body and mind. Choose from lemon oil that cleanses and detoxifies;

lavender comforts and relaxes; eucalyptus aids in respiration; ginger stimulates and warms.

Yoga–The Perfect Balance

Yoga creates a balanced and whole-hearted acceptance of life at this phase of life when kids are moving on to make their own life and you are left alone when you need them most. A sense of loneliness sets in, when earlier your life revolved around the family. This is the time to spend on your own self, if all these years you have neglected yourself. This is the time to connect with your true self, do things that you always wanted to do, go on a hike, spend time with Nature, learn the salsa and simply love and take care of yourself. Yoga and meditation will teach you to accept the present as it is and teach you to live life with awareness. It will teach you to stay grounded and centred even if life is full of changes. A consistent practice of yoga will help you move in the direction of deeper appreciation of life and take you away from the unending struggles and dissatisfaction. Yoga will create within you the feeling of contentment and fill your inner being with tranquillity and peace.

Yoga–A Spiritual Practice

Karma yoga is a path of selflessness through serving and working without desiring an end reward. *Bhakti* yoga is worship of the Divine and is the path of devotion, usually practiced by chanting prayers and *mantras*. *Jnana* yoga is the study of the self, spiritual scriptures and the Divine. It is an intellectual approach to spiritual evolution.

Raja yoga is a scientific and a systematic path of analysis in meditation, that helps to erase ego and to dissolve it with the thinking mind into oneness.

All these paths can be combined in your *hatha* yoga, to deepen the practice and spiritual connection.